Table of Contents

I0435681

Introduction

Floods have been one of the major natural catastrophes, which mankind has had to survive through the millenniums. Since prehistoric times, he knew that there were going to be occasions, when suddenly powerful spates of water would come churning down mountains, sweeping everything before them.

The rains which affected mankind 7000 years ago, for 40 days and 40 nights must have brought its accompanying floods, which wiped out a large percentage of mankind. However, there were still survivors, those who got to other lands and raise their families there. These tales of the great floods have been a historic part and parcel of historic knowledge passed down the generations since the times of Gilgamesh.

Even all these millenniums later, mankind is still vulnerable to floods, but with a little bit of technological know-how, and a little bit of preparedness, he can save his family from total disaster. Remember that this is the 21st century, and anybody who is under the impression that This Thing Cannot Happen to Me, is living in a fool's paradise.

We may be better prepared to survive, with State and Center rescue programs started up by our local armies, or our governments, to take care of us in case of a flood, but even those are not completely hundred percent effective and reliable, especially the weather is inclement.

Survival of the fittest means that many people would rather be safe than sorry, and these includes people of rescue groups, working on flood disaster management and rescue.

A Beginner's Guide to Flood Survival

Flood Survival Tips and Techniques

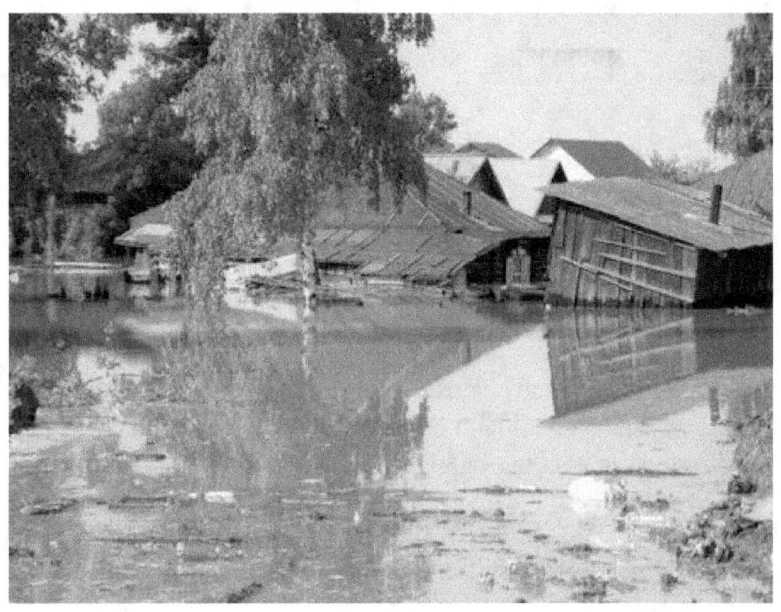

Prepping and Survival Book Series

Dueep J. Singh

Mendon Cottage Books

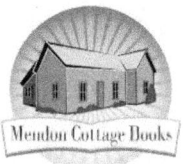

JD-Biz Publishing

Disclaimer

The information is this book is provided for informational purposes only. It is not intended to be used and medical advice or a substitute for proper medical treatment by a qualified health care provider. The information is believed to be accurate as presented based on research by the author.

The contents have not been evaluated by the U.S. Food and Drug Administration or any other Government or Health Organization and the contents in this book are not to be used to treat cure or prevent disease.

The author or publisher is not responsible for the use or safety of any diet, procedure or treatment mentioned in this book. The author or publisher is not responsible for errors or omissions that may exist.

Warning

The Book is for informational purposes only and before taking on any diet, treatment or medical procedure, it is recommended to consult with your primary health care provider.

Check out some of the other Healthy Gardening Series books at Amazon.com

Gardening Series on Amazon

Check out some of the other Health Learning Series books at Amazon.com

Health Learning Series on Amazon

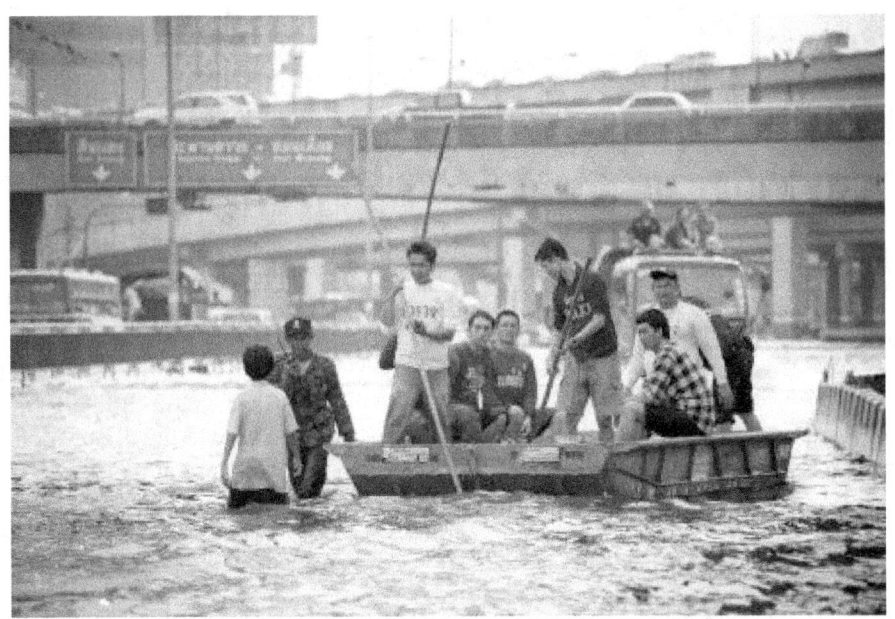

It may take a while for the authorities to get to you, so until then, you need to survive.

Flood survival can be implemented with a little bit of basic common sense. As this natural calamity is one of the problems affecting mankind, globally, man, through experience, has begun to understand times when places are going to flood and he has been protecting himself down the centuries during such times.

The ancient Egyptians knew all about the flooding of the Nile at periodic intervals, and they had the good sense not to build their cities in the areas, where those floods occurred ever so often. Instead, they made sure that they moved their families to higher ground, during those flooding seasons, and spent those months building pyramids for their Pharaoh. The Cecil B. DeMille visualization of the pyramids made by slaves under the supervision of cruel whip cracking overseers is pure fantasy.

Egyptians – workers, farmers and freeborn Egyptians – were proud to lend a hand in making these large objects of Egypt's glory, during times, when they could not work in the fields. This labor was purely voluntary and well, these farmers and workers, helping to build the pyramids, were given bread and onions to eat, after a hard day's work. And so the pyramids were raised.

I would not be surprised if somewhere, some excavator may come up with some Egyptian hieroglyphics , saying "Soser of XYZ village helped in the building of this pyramid, during the annual flooding of the Nile in the year ..."

And then after the flooding was over, they went back to their villages, and raised their crops on the rich and fertile soil, brought to their land by the waters of the river. So the natural circle of water evaporation, cloud formation and rains – possibly heavy rain, leading to floods – is going to be an integral part of human life as long as he lives on this earth.

As this natural circle is ordained, you cannot change it. However, a little bit of preparedness, tips and techniques to survive floods, and knowledge about food and water, which you need to have around you to keep you healthy, when your land has been flooded out should be learned right now in your flood disaster management arsenal of knowledge.

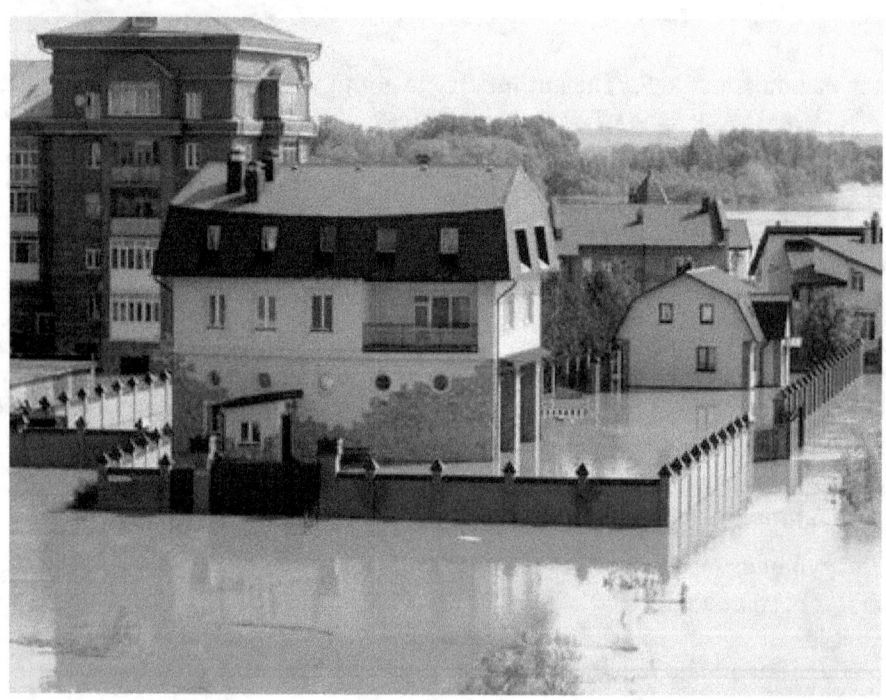

So like the Boy Scouts, Be Prepared.

Types of Flooding

There are two types of flooding, which one normally sees in nature. The "normal" flooding is going to be periodic, which may occur after a heavy or a long period of rains. That is because that area is prone to floods. It can also be caused due to the melting of the snow in the mountains and the ensuing water coming down the slopes to the plains overfilling the rivers.

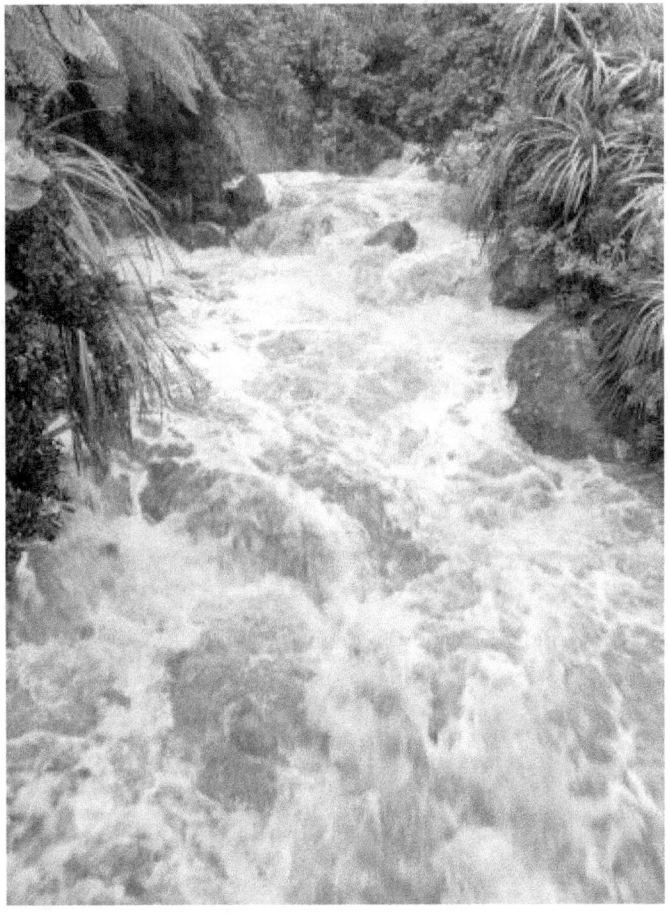

Flash floods are more dangerous than seasonal floods

21st century man is going to be susceptible to more and more incidents of this type of flooding, as global warming causes more snow to melt in the mountains.

Also, the melting of the ice caps in the Arctic regions has raised the level of the water in the sea. This water evaporates, and is going to make more clouds which are going to burst into heavy rainfall, all over the land. And that is going to cause flooding. The floodwater is going to evaporate soon,   make more clouds, and then precipitate again into more floods.

Man cannot do anything about it, because he has already started up this vicious chain of a Catch-22 situation. That is why nearly every year, we hear about water levels in rivers and creeks rising because of this extra runoff of water, until you have water covering the land, or just going over the banks in an overflow.

Along with this normal flooding, there is another natural catastrophe, pertaining to flowing water – flash floods. These are more dangerous, because they can occur anywhere, anytime, and hit with little warning. Flash floods can cover an area in just seconds, and destroy everything before them.

I know about a family who is living in an area prone to flash floods. They have been flooded out many times. Being of a practical nature, I asked them whether it was not more sensible if they left that area and settled somewhere where it was comparatively safe. The answer they gave me was that their ancestors had been living in that area for millenniums, and they had no intention of moving.

Well, if you have no intention of moving, it is much better to that you use a little bit of common sense to save you and your family during a rainstorm.

I would suggest that you do not relax and sleep during a heavy rain storm. That is because a flash flood can occur anytime, and you may not have another chance to take your family to safety if you are busy hunting for your shoes. Debris and water coming down in force during a rainstorm can cause instant disaster.

Safety Tips – before a Flood

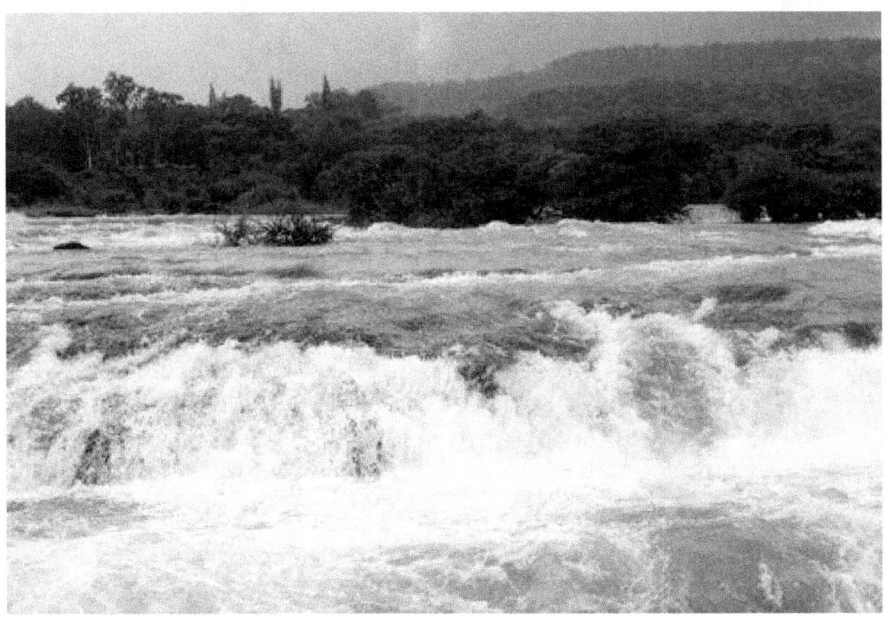

Unregulated water let free through a dam can cause flash floods

I spent a major part of my life as a child and then as an adult, moving from place to place, in a transferable job. The first thing I used to ask when I got my transfer orders was – how far was it from the sea, the coastal area, rivers, and was that area prone to floods? After that, I would take measures to counteract a flood situation if it ever occurred. It never did.

Call this distrustful behavior, but then, anybody who has already been through flood water –literally - as a nine-year-old child and has been swept away by a raging river – the river Tunghabhadra in the South of India [*I came, I saw, I slipped on a rock, I fell*]-is going to be wary about the power of water. That river is flooded yearly with seasonal rains from the monsoon.

I was rescued by someone grabbing my hair and pulling me out. I would not be here writing this, if fate had not brought that hefty quick thinking good Samaritan on the bank of the river that morning. You may not be so lucky.

Luckily, most of the time, I was posted to desert or dry plain areas, so I did not have to worry about normal flooding. But flash floods can happen anytime and that is why we never made our camps in what we could see were dried riverbeds. Why take a chance?

Somebody may tell you, that this is a desert area, and it has not rained here for 20 years, but Murphy's Law is always applicable where I am concerned. So if you know that an area has been flooded during the last couple of years, there is a chance that it is going to be vulnerable to flooding this year too.

That is because the geography of the land has not changed and history is going to repeat itself as nature asserts herself every year. Also, the land can also change its topological nature through the shifting of its underground tectonic plates due to possible underground earthquakes. That means any source of water, which is underground can come up to the surface and vice versa.

There are very few places all over the earth which are not vulnerable to possible floods. Dams may check the spate of the river, but in many cases, they are not very effective, especially when they have been damaged due to the power of water, down the years. So a dam burst means an even greater catastrophe.

Living in a Flood Prone Area

If you are living in an area which is prone to normal floods, keep all your important belongings and possessions on the second or third floor of your house. That means if your ground-floor is flooded out, you will suffer from water damage, but most of your belongings are going to be safe. Of course, this rule is not going to be worth a red cent, if your house is swept away in a flash flood.

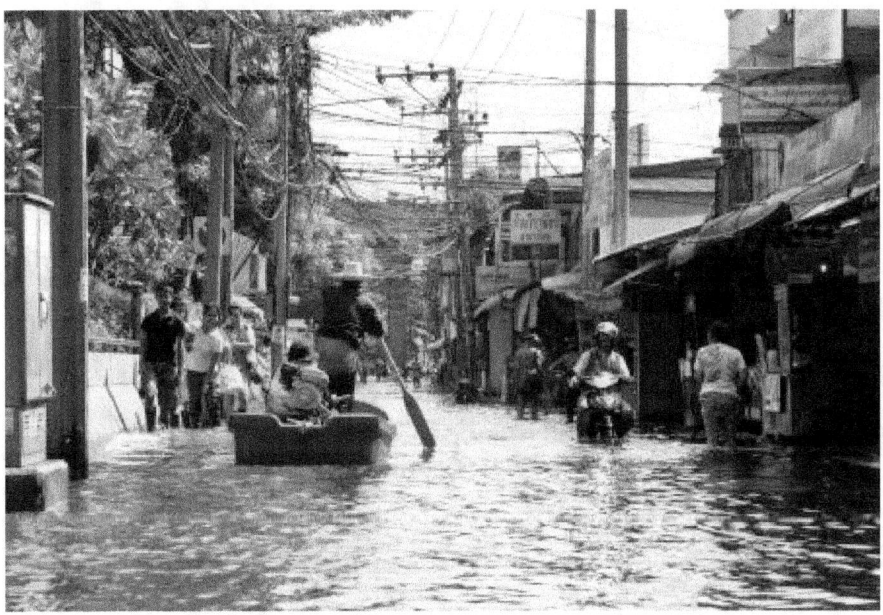

The moment your area is affected by a flood, you are going to find the basic amenities being turned off. That means you may not have access to water and electricity. This is when you had to take full advantage of a flood survival kit.

Survival Kit

According to the American Red Cross, these are the items you need to have easily accessible. It is suggested that you keep these kits handy, at home, or which you can take with you if you need to evacuate.

These are the minimum items which you need to keep you and your family safe.

A three-day supply of water in case of evacuation, and two week supply for home use. 1 gallon of water per person/per day should be stored.

Food – a two week supply of easy to prepare, and nonperishable items for home use, and four days' supply in case of evacuation.

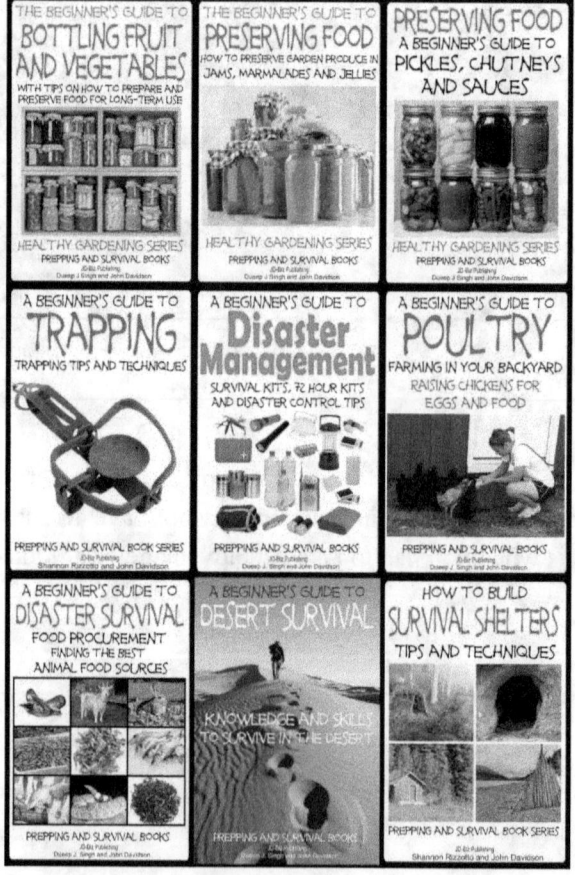

A multipurpose tool, especially a Swiss Army knife is always handy. Along with that, you need a good sturdy flashlight, batteries – rechargeable batteries are not going to do here, because you may not have access to electricity – and a handcranked radio.

Necessary medical items, and medication.

The size of the kit is going to depend upon the size of your family. So, look at this list of items placed in your own personalized survival kit and start ticking your list.

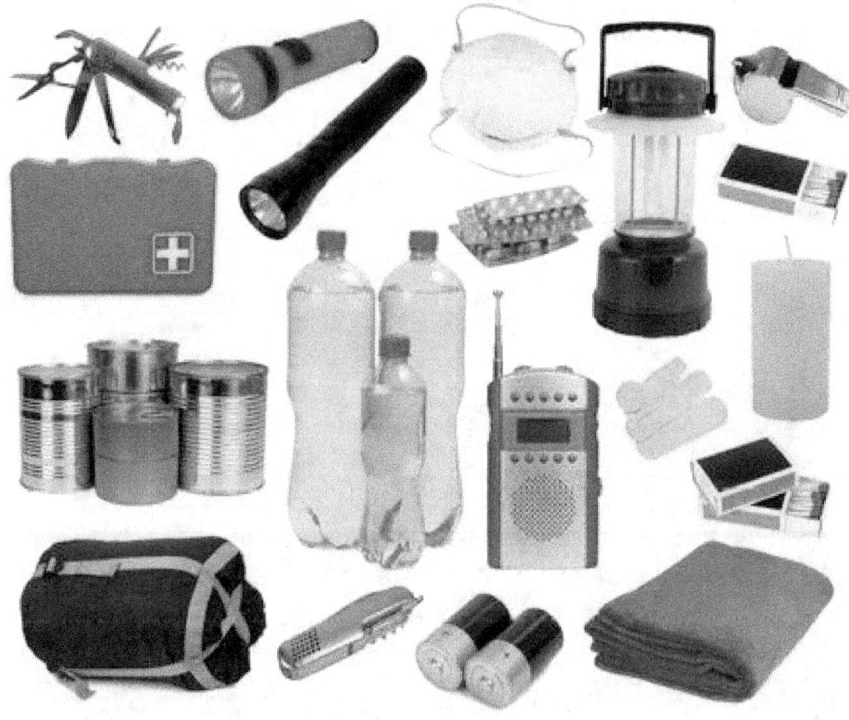

For Warmth and Shelter

Clothes, according to the weather, lightweight rain guard, tube tent, lightweight space blanket for warmth, heavy gloves and shoes.

Magnifying glass for lighting fires, waterproof matches, lighter, and butane fuel, and torches with battery. You can also add PLBs (personal locator beacon), candles, flashlights, compasses, paper and pens, and a map for signaling purposes to the kit.

Your first aid kit is going to have sterile gauze, bandages and first aid tape, scissors, disinfectants, Ibuprofen and oxytetracycline. Include soap, feminine personal hygiene products and insect repellent.

The important first-aid supplies include antiseptic creams and sprays, burn ointment, tweezers and a micropore bandage sticking plaster roll, which can be cut without the help of scissors.

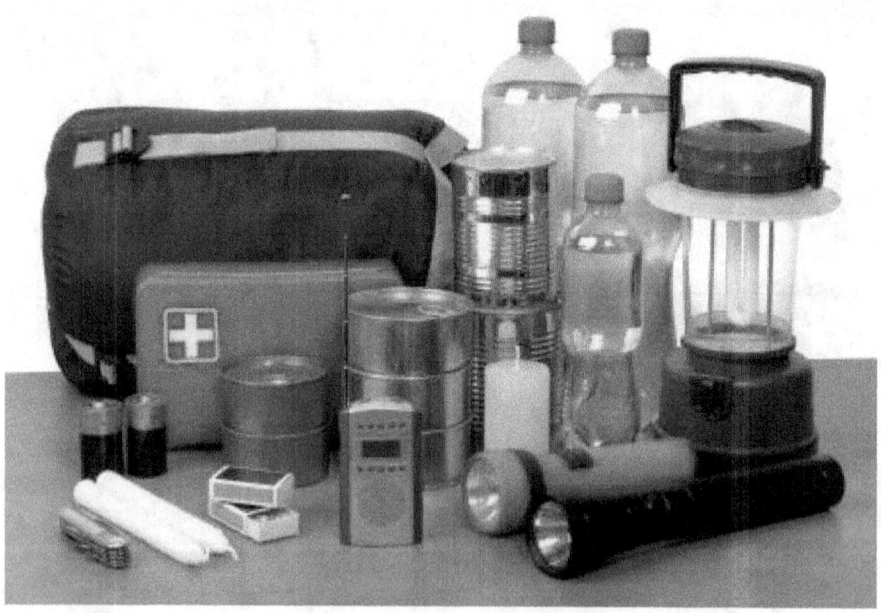

72 Hour survival Kit

Food and water for a 72 hour kit includes water purifying iodine tablets and salt for food, canned foods, tin opener and fishing tools.

Sleeping bags for every family member, extra clothes, both for winter and for summer, blankets, canvas shoes (keds) and socks, water purifying tablets, flashlights with battery, personal hygiene products, rainproof bedding and covering, high calorie long lasting food bars, flashlights, multipurpose knife and easily ignited fuel tablets, along with a lighter are just some of the important things which need to be added to your survival kit.

Some people also put in portable radios with a long-lasting battery in the kit.

A good survival kit can be considered to be a 72 hour kit, because you need to suppose yourself cut away from rescue operations in about this time limit. This is of course the worst-case scenario, but 3 days is the bare minimum of time for which you need to be prepared.

Medical prescriptions, along with the dosage as well as important family papers, like certificates, passports, driving license, etc. can also be stored away in the survival kits. Also put in some ready cash and credit cards in the kit.

Now you need to look at the water supply. Each family member needs at least one gallon of water, every day. So you need easy access to stored water, kept away from the sunlight.

Along with these items, make sure that you have personal hygiene items and sanitation items, including a comb. I have found that just combing your hair when you are stressed out, sort of relaxes you, because not only are you going back to your mode of – I am well groomed, I am in control, but it makes you feel good. That is the reason why prisoners of war officers suffering in prison camps always made sure that they never slipped into the mode of slip shoddy clothing or personal appearance.

One, it was a matter of pride, two, it was to keep their own morale high, even though their circumstances and surroundings were pitiful and pathetic.

Even though the American Red Cross asks you keep your working cell phone with the charger in your survival kit, you may consider it an extra. It is not going to be of any use, if there is no network and no electricity to charge your cell phone. So you find yourself with a useless piece of machinery on your hands.

Make sure that your family has emergency information, with contact numbers, identification marks, blood group and medical allergies written carefully in documents which they are going to carry all the while. This is in case you get separated, and someone needs to know their identities.

A good map of the area should begin to everybody and map training should be done with all your family members so that they know where they are and where they need to go in cases of emergency.

Hearing aids and other battery operated aids should have extra batteries. Also, have extra pairs of glasses and contact lenses added to your survival kit.

If there is a baby in the family, you need to have enough of baby supplies, including diapers, baby formula, baby bottles and baby food. Same thing goes for pets – leash, carrier, collar and bowls along with food. Though often, pets are discarded on the roadside, in a mad scramble to save oneself. It is *sauve qui peut* in many cases, especially when the mind is still shocked in the aftermath of a catastrophe.

Every family member should have an extra pair of house keys and car keys. You may also want 2 way walkie-talkies or radios with extra batteries.

All right, that reminds me. Make sure that you have a number of can openers and knives, if you are waiting for rescue at home. Can openers have this bad habit of disappearing when you need them most. I had three, and never could find them, especially when I needed to open up bottles and cans, real fast. Even hanging them in prominent places in the kitchen did not work. They went walkabout ever so often.

So I tried another idea – a key ring to which a bottle/can opener is attached. And as I do not lose my keys so often, I know where I can get the bottle/can opener ready at hand.

Apart from this, other survival gear can include plenty of towels, an emergency police whistle, a paraffin stove with paraffin, emergency police whistle, good lighter because even waterproof matches get lost when you need them, plenty of candles, and supplies and tools to repair and secure your home.

These tools are going to include sharp scissors, duct tape, screwdrivers, hammers and nails. Look for manual tools, because in the paucity of electricity, electric drills and other electricity operated tools are not going to work at all.

This is, of course, when we are looking at the worst-case scenario.

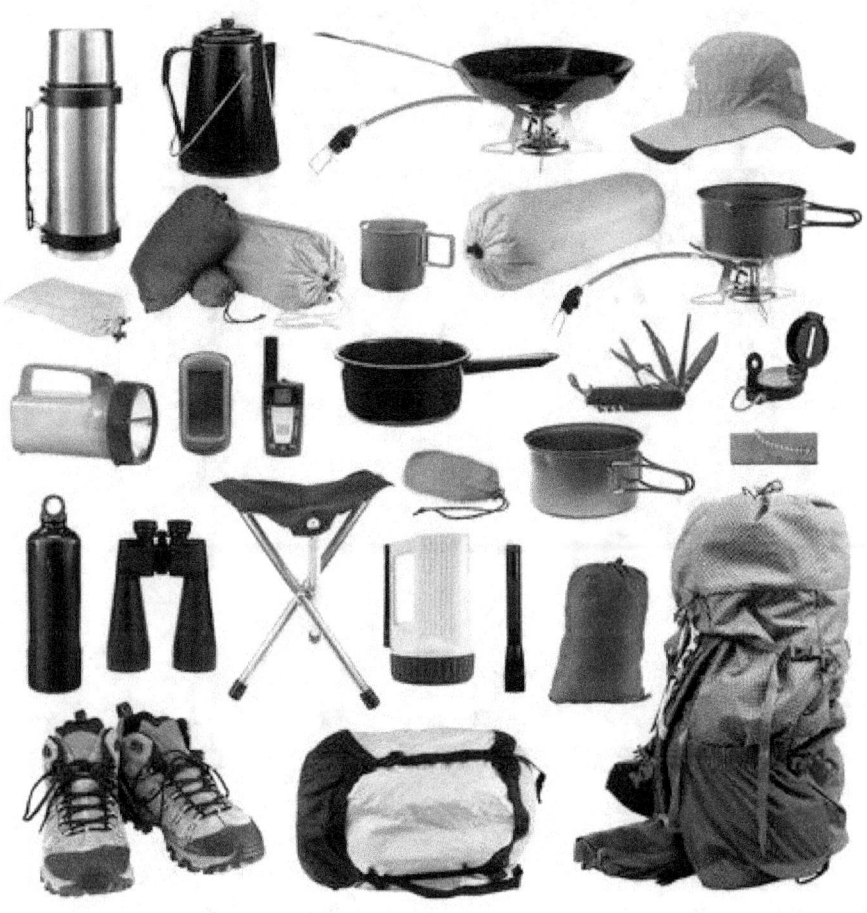

What to Do during a Flood

Just imagine that your area has been flooded. Do not immediately get into your car and tried to drive away. This is dangerous for you and your family. 6 inches of water on the road is going to stall your car and there you are, you cannot get anywhere.

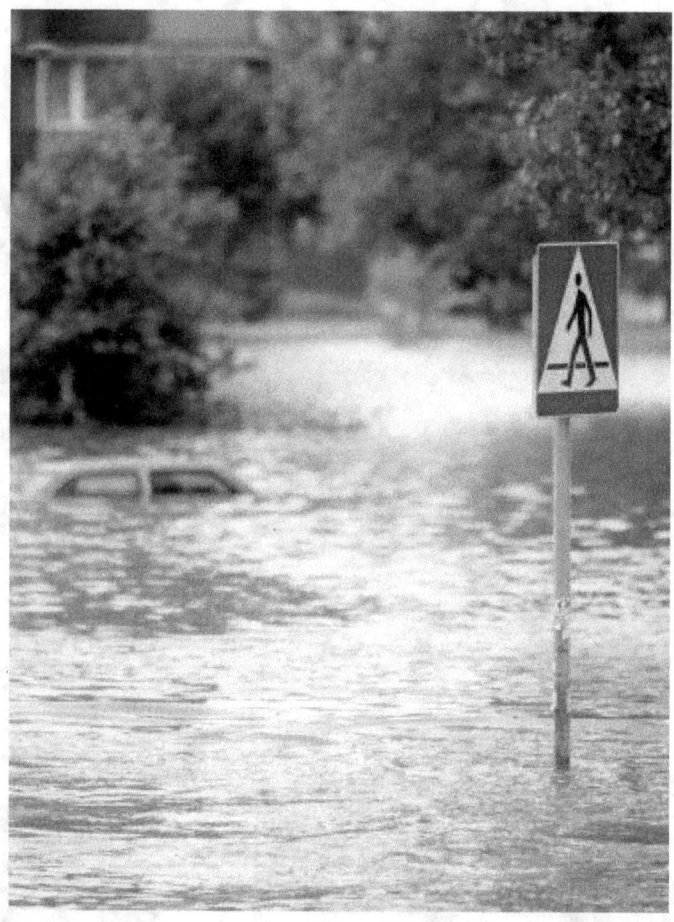

Also, driving on wet roads is definitely not advised. That is because the surface is slippery and treacherous and can cause your car to skid. Also, if you do not know how deep the water level is on the road and you cannot see it, how do you know that you are driving on the road and not into an open drain or gutter?

In the 90s, I remember living in a neighborhood which used to get flooded out periodically every year with the coming of the rains. And as I needed to get to my office by walking through water, in order to reach the Metro, – no driving – I used to ask the people who had been living in that area, how to get through 18-25 inches of water without disappearing into *an open drain.*

Yes, there are still neighborhoods and places where the drains are left open in our towns and cities.

And they used to tell me, just hug the walls, and clutch them when you are walking to the Metro. Do not walk where you think the road used to be, because we do not know whether it is there or not! Also, I needed to hold onto a rope strung from one end of the walls to the other, and not move an inch away from the rope, because even 16 inches of swirling twirling water would be enough to make me lose my footing and get ducked in floodwater.

Also, I needed to step wary, because no one knew what hazardous pieces of debris were hiding underground waiting to hurt my legs and shins wading through the water.

 So, not being a sensible person, I used to roll up my uniform trousers to mid-thigh, tie my socks and shoes around my neck, take a pair of rubber slippers out of my briefcase,-rubber waders and galoshes would have been waterlogged immediately – put my faith in God and go wading through deep and dank muddy water, where once there was land.

This is not an unusual occurrence in the life and times of people living in the East, especially during the rains! We go with the flow, no pun intended. Also, when I reached my destination, my acquaintances would ask me whether their stalled cars were still safe and sound, – in the water where they had been left or not? – That is how the stalled car network works.

Now, I would not advise you to do this, because I was going through rainwater, which had not been drained away. Floodwater is going to have dangerous debris, and even venomous snakes and insects in it. So, under no circumstances, walk, or wade through flood water, unless absolutely necessary. I had to, like the rest of my fellow citizens, because this was a yearly occurrence, until I was transferred elsewhere. But this is definitely not a sensible procedure.

I did not suffer from skin diseases due to exposure to this contaminated water, because the moment I used to reach my destination, I used to scrub me under a shower with water and antiseptic. So God does take care of fools, often.

There was also one other potential hazard, of which I knew nothing when wading through this water. Underground electric cables, and live ones. They would have roasted me alive. These are potential dangers of which you should know when the floods come in.

If I had any sense, I would have taken a stick to probe for underground obstacles, and even open drains, especially if I needed to walk in the middle of nowhere where I thought there was a road under all that slow flowing water. So like I said, if you have to go into water, carry a stick to prod and "see" where you are going to put your next foot.

What If You Are on the Road in a Flood Situation?

Like I said, never drive when you are going through floods. But what if you find yourself on the road, and there is flood water everywhere? So stop your vehicle and try to get to a relatively dry area. You can always come back and rescue your vehicle, but if the floodwater swirls you away, trapped inside your vehicle, you are going to be one of the statistics of this year's floods.

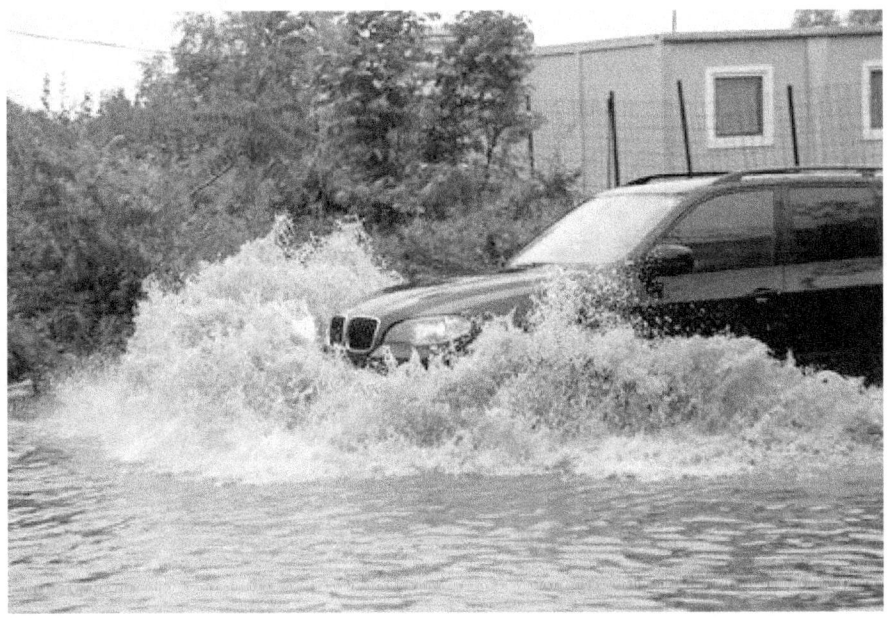

Big mistake…

Also, take the advice of more sensible people, if you really have to cross an area which has been flooded. About four decades ago, father with his bride was driving to his Base, only to find that the road had been flooded a couple of days previously.

He knew where the road was. But his instinct told him, stop, and wait till he saw another driver.

10 minutes later he heard a truck driver yelling at him in the native vernacular, something on the lines of "hey, thou *Sahib* with thy car, thou follow me. I will take thee and thine to safety. "

That burly truck driver drove 5 miles down the road and crossed the waters there. When father thanked him and asked him why people were not crossing the road at the previous location, he was told that there was a 25 feet deep hole, where once there was a road.

So if father had taken a chance and gone through the water, he, my future mother, and their car would have disappeared into that hole and with no one knowing what happened to them, ever. So never take a chance.

Preventing Water Contamination

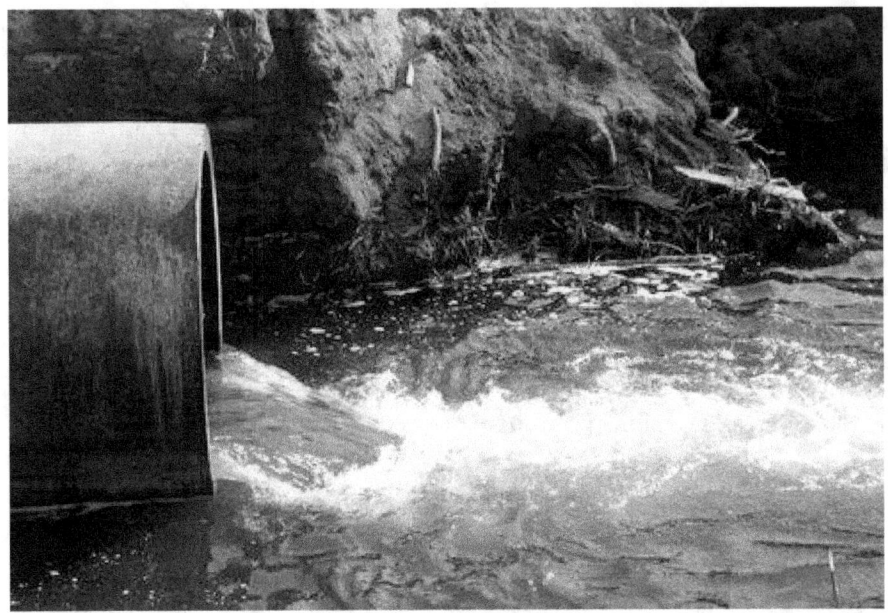

All this debris is going to cause contamination of water after a flood

Water contamination is one of the hazards which you will have to face in case of floods. That is because dirty water from external sources like rain or the river is going to mix up with your normal water source. That means immediate pollution, especially if this contamination means River water being mixed up with drinking water.

Everyone knows that all the rivers in the world are absolutely filthy with chemical and industrial waste. When this water gets mixed up with your drinking water, you have had it.

So every drop of water which you are going to drink during a flood situation has to be boiled and filtered. If you already have your pure water containers ready at hand, that is good, because that is the water that you are going to be using for drinking purposes.

But if you are taking water from some other outer source, never drink it straight from the tap or any other water source. Consider that to be a potential health hazard and boil and filter it.

Do the water filtering tablets work? Yes, they do, but boiling and filtering is also more efficient because that is going to kill the germs and straining that boiled water is going to get rid of any potential debris, dust, dirt, or extra bits of material in the water.

If the water is contaminated by chemicals and Sewage, you are going to suffer from skin diseases and epidemics. Why are doctors so scared after a flood? They know that the percentage of survivors who are going to succumb to a water borne disease is going to be very high, because many people do not bother about ingesting contaminated water.

In the olden days, the Kings of South India used to protect their land from flood waters by flood proofing the banks with sandbags, walls and trees. We can still find those vestiges of flood proofing barriers there today.

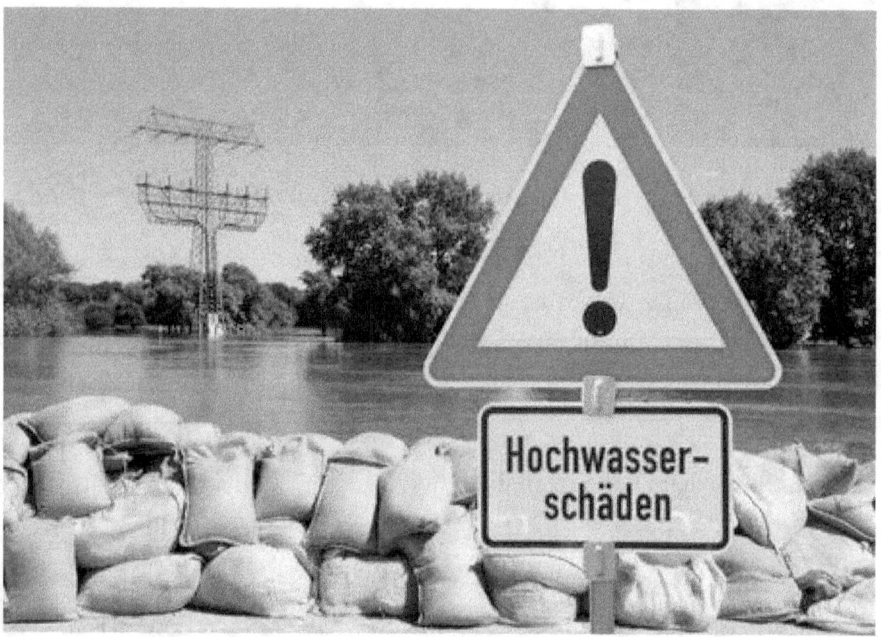

Flood prone countries in Europe are using this method to prevent their land from being flooded. You can do the same by protecting your property with these flood barriers. Apart from sandbags and stonewalls, you can also use lumber.
Remember that floods are a natural powerful force of nature. But you can lessen its power and intensity by using these barriers.

Precautions When Confronted with a Flood

If you find you in a house, trapped in a flood here are some things which you do not do. Do not use any electrical appliances because any sort of electric leakage is going to cause an accident. Instead, it is more sensible to turn off all the electricity supply from the mains, as well as the gas supply so that there is no gas leakage either.

Fill all the water containers with clean water, and then cut off the water supply so that you do not get contaminated water flowing in your water pipes. All of these supplies are going to be switched off from the main shutoff points, so you should know where they are, you should know how to operate them, and you should have easy access to them when in case of emergency.

If you can, try to get out of the house, to an area where it is comparatively dry. One does not try to swim in any sort of flood water, because not only is this not safe, but it is also potentially life-threatening and dangerous. Especially, when the water is flowing swiftly, and there are currents of floodwater.

Make sure that none of your family members are near electric lines or electric appliances.

If You Are Outdoors during a Flood

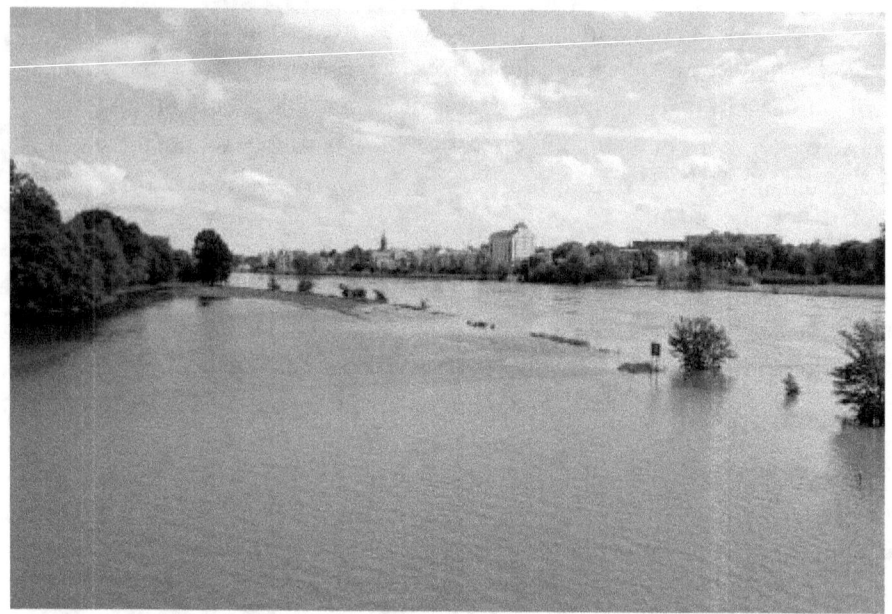

If you find you outdoors, especially during vacation times, and you get a message that there is a chance of your area being flooded in the near future, keep a lookout at the weather. Get your family to higher ground, because when the floods come you are not going to have any chance to think logically and at a leisurely pace.

Remember that Hurry, worry and scurry always ruins the curry, so flapping around and wringing your hands, saying, *what are we going to do what are we going to do* is not going to help matters. When we are talking about clichés, God helps those who help themselves, so do not keep waiting for somebody else to come to help you. Use your brains and your common sense.

Do not go driving out of the city, trying to escape the flood because you do not know when it is going to appear and from which direction. And if you find yourself trapped along with your family in a car, and being swept away with flood waters, you are definitely going to be in dire straits.

Also, many people have a tendency of leaving a disaster area, in a panic, especially when they have left the evacuation to the last moment. Human beings have a tendency of saying, "this cannot happen to us," even though it has been proven that this has happened every year and this is going to happen every year, but most of us will never learn.

We will go back to the flood area, which was flooded out a couple of months ago, and start building again in that particular area. And when we are asked to evacuate, we are more worried about our property instead of our lives.

I have seen that, especially when I was a part of a flood evacuation team, going along with state administrators to get people out of vulnerable villages in the Eastern parts of the country, where floods are part of everyday life, every year.

I was confronted by stubborn villagers who would not move. When I asked the district authorities what they did, under such circumstances, they said that the world was full of fools, born fools and stubborn fools. One could do absolutely nothing about such people. It is a well-known fact that people evacuated from a danger zone crept back at night to their homes, because that was the only area where they felt safe. And they died there.

But as this book is being read by a person who is sensible, and who knows the importance of checking on weather report and weather watch stations, and then taking proper measures to ensure the security of family and self, I know that these tips which are being given in this book are going to be implemented in cases of flood.

So if you are outside, in a vehicle and you find flood waters appearing, just strap on your survival kit bag on your back and get to higher ground as fast as possible. Do not go back to the vehicle, saying that you want to save your collection of CDs or your video games. Firstly, what makes you think that these video games and CDs are absolutely necessary for your survival, especially when food, water and shelter are your first priority.

Why did I say the above statement about inessential things? Because I saw a flood victim running back into a potentially dangerous zone, because she wanted to get her jewelry box and makeup kit. For her, those were absolutely important items, necessary for her survival. If she believed that, she should have put it in her survival kit. Seriously, I would suggest that if you have precious items you want protected, put them in a safer location away from the flood zone. If you have to carry them with you, stitch them into your clothing.

After A Flood – Your Personal Safety

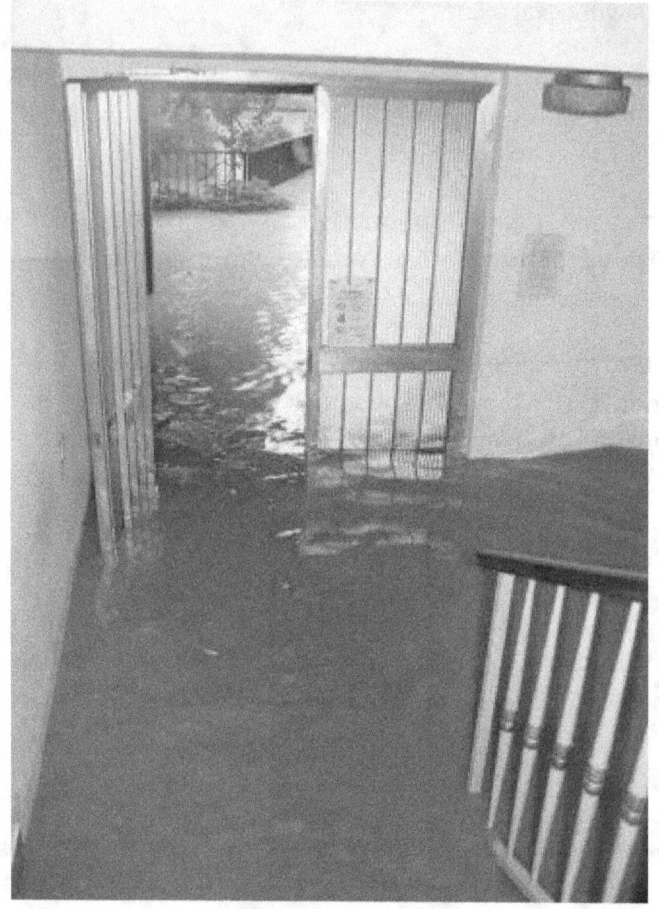

Do not go running back into a damaged area, trying to assess the damage after the floods have gone down. Most of us do that without bothering about the authorities checking whether it is safe to go there or not. That is man's natural instinct to make sure that his property is intact and that the two legged vultures accompanying the rescue teams after any catastrophe have not rummaged through that damaged area in search of valuables.

This unfortunately is also a part of the tragedy of natural catastrophes. Since 2013, a particular area of the Indian subcontinent has been subjected to landslides, floods and other natural catastrophes before the rainy season and during a time, when pilgrims go to the mountains on a pilgrimage.

The authorities cannot prevent the pilgrims from not going into the danger zone because religion is a very touchy subject all over the world. Also, pilgrims cannot be persuaded not to do something, when they have decided that they need to go on pilgrimage starting from March. And when the rains come down and the landslides cause pieces of mountains to break away, literally thousands are swept away. The Army and the Air Force is then called in to rescue the stranded pilgrims and hunt for survivors.

After the catastrophe is over, it is then the job of these men and other law enforcing authorities to round up all those thieves who plunder and pillage the dead bodies of their valuables. Last year, gold and jewels worth $30 million and more were confiscated from these vultures. But then this is human nature, because down the centuries, this has taken place.

After the battle of Waterloo, the bodies of dead and dying soldiers were stripped of every valuable, and even articles of clothing, so that many people who could have survived froze to death. So this is where I talk about personal safety. Have a firearm close to you, to protect you and your family.

But I believe in nonviolence, you may say. I hate firearms or weapons of violence. Well, if you would rather have your children being injured by people who want to take away their survival packs from them, just because you are too timid to try to protect them, well, that is your outlook. And also remember that it is of no use, just waving a firearm and threatening to use it. You should have the mental strength to use it when necessary. This is of course not possible by many of us who deplore the idea of violence.

But if you do not have the will to survive, you had better believe in the fatalistic idea of "what will be will be, and if it has been fated for my children to be hurt by undisciplined gangs, "that is your prerogative.

But I have noticed that this is more of an Eastern concept. The Westerners are tougher, there will to survive is stronger and they do not give up easily. That is because they know that sitting and moaning is not going to help them, but decisive and strong action is going to get them out of dire situations.

I enjoy reading Peter O'Donnell's Modesty Blaise, because of one statement he made about her creation. "She does not give up even when the knife is at her throat. As long as she has one breath of life in her, she is going to look for a way to survive and cheat death. And she does. "Modesty is definitely not fatalistic!

Fatalism is in my opinion the easiest resort for a person who is not willing to make any sort of effort in anything ever, in life, – and taking a flood situation into account, – and in possible death.

When should you start removing the floodwater from your property? Once it has been deemed to be safe by the authorities will have checked up that there are no live electricity lines, take the help of experts, especially flood inspectors.

They are going to visit your property and assess the amount of damage done, for insurance purposes, as well as for calculating rebuilding expenses. Trying to remove the floodwater on your own can damage the property even more.

Also, remember not to drink the tap water, which has been switched on after a flood has affected the area, for a couple of days. Still continue drinking the boiled water. Also, any food, fruit or vegetable, which has come through flood water – if raw – needs to be washed properly before you eat it.

If you have built a house in a flood prone area, remember to construct it on a higher level, so that it is comparatively safe from flooding. The electric panel, electric furnace and heater should be built at a height, so that floodwaters do not reach them.

Floodwalls and beams are barriers which can prevent flood damage. Also, make sure that your plumbing, especially the sewer traps have check valves, which means that any sort of floodwater is not going to drain into your home's drainage system.

Seepage in constructions built underground can be prevented by using waterproofing materials and compounds for sealing and construction.

If you get a warning of a flash flood in your area, take immediate steps and moved to a higher area. Do not keep waiting for orders from the authority to evacuate. They imagine and hope that you have the instinct and common sense to protect yourself and your family.

But before you leave your house, you need to secure it. Move all the essential items to a higher level in your house. Turn off all the valves and switches, including the water and electricity supplies.

Never touch any electrical appliance if the floor is wet or you are standing in floodwater.

While walking to a higher ground, carry a sturdy stick along with your survival pack. Naturally, you are going to be wearing sensible and sturdy long-lasting shoes, protective clothing – comfortable trousers and loose shirts. Have a number of changes of clothing in your survival pack, because you may have need of dry clothing.

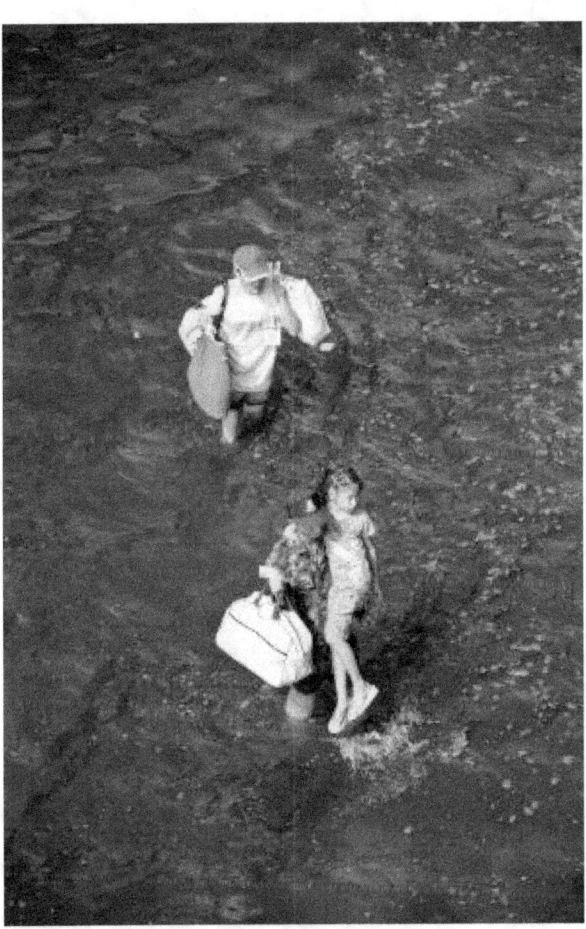

Driving After a Flood

Make sure that any area which was covered by floodwater and where the waters have receded now is safe to travel. That is because the area may have grown weak. And if you are driving over it, it may collapse.

Floodwater is going to be contaminated with chemicals and gasoline. So not only is it toxic, but you have to make sure that you do not expose your body to it.

Flooding and Insurance

Many insurance companies do not cover flood damage, under normal homeowners policies, so you need to make sure that your insurance company gives you a policy, under which you can ensure your house and its items against potential flood damage on hazards.

You may want to talk to any reliable and experienced insurance agent who will help you get the best flood insurance policy. It takes about 30 days for your policy to get activated, in America, so act right now and protect your home against floods.

If your insurance agent told you that he cannot offer you a flood insurance policy, because you are living in a flood prone zone, change your agent! Flood insurance is readily available regardless of whether your property is within or outside a possible flood prone area.

Conclusion

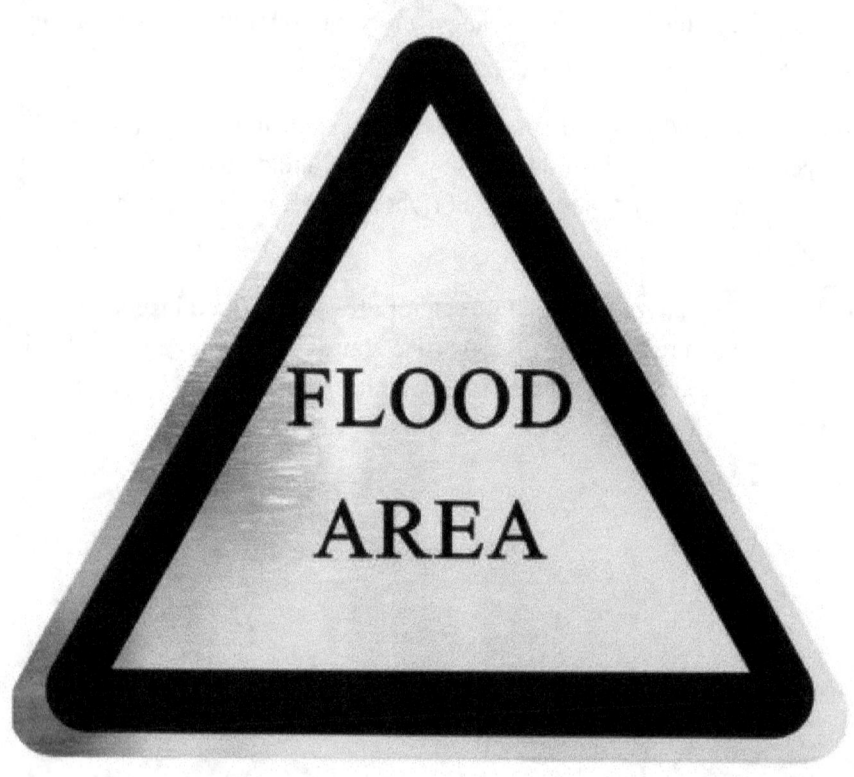

This book in our disaster management series has given you a number of tips about what to do when you are subject to a flood. Remember that any natural catastrophe is going to be accompanied with personal mental, spiritual, emotional and physical tension and trauma, especially when you are not ready for it.

But mankind has been surviving these catastrophes for millenniums. It is a measure of his strength and willpower, which makes him bounce back and carry on, even though he has gone through desperate moments when he thinks that all is lost.

I am not going to use clichés here and say trite aphorisms. But when a person is called upon to survive, he is going to find the will to do so, especially when his instinct puts the well-being of his family first.

So Live Long and Prosper! And keep safe with the tips and tricks given in our disaster management series – available right here.

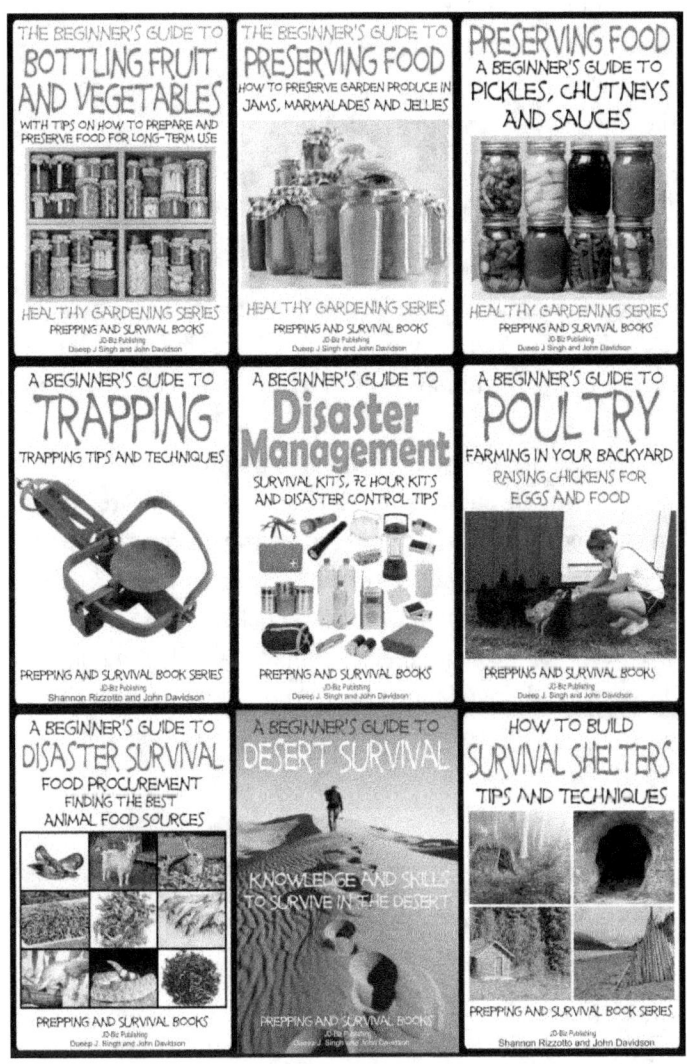

Author Bio

Dueep Jyot Singh is a Management and IT Professional who managed to gather Postgraduate qualifications in Management and English and Degrees in Science, French and Education while pursuing different enjoyable career options like being an hospital administrator, IT,SEO and HRD Database Manager/ trainer, movie , radio and TV scriptwriter, theatre artiste and public speaker, lecturer in French, Marketing and Advertising, ex-Editor of Hearts On Fire (now known as Solstice) Books Missouri USA, advice columnist and cartoonist, publisher and Aviation School trainer, ex- moderator on Medico.in, banker, student councilor ,travelogue writer … among other things!

One fine morning, she decided that she had enough of killing herself by Degrees and went back to her first love -- writing. It's more enjoyable! She already has 48 published academic and 14 fiction- in- different- genre books under her belt.

When she is not designing websites or making Graphic design illustrations for clients , she is browsing through old bookshops hunting for treasures, of which she has an enviable collection – including R.L. Stevenson, O.Henry, Dornford Yates, Maurice Walsh, De Maupassant, Victor Hugo, Sapper, C.N. Williamson, "Bartimeus" and the crown of her collection- Dickens "The Old Curiosity Shop," and so on… Just call her "Renaissance Woman") - collecting herbal remedies, acting like Universal Helping Hand/Agony Aunt, or escaping to her dear mountains for a bit of exploring, collecting herbs and plants and trekking.

Our books are available at

1. Amazon.com
2. Barnes and Noble
3. Itunes
4. Kobo
5. Smashwords
6. Google Play Books

Check out some of the other JD-Biz Publishing books

Gardening Series on Amazon

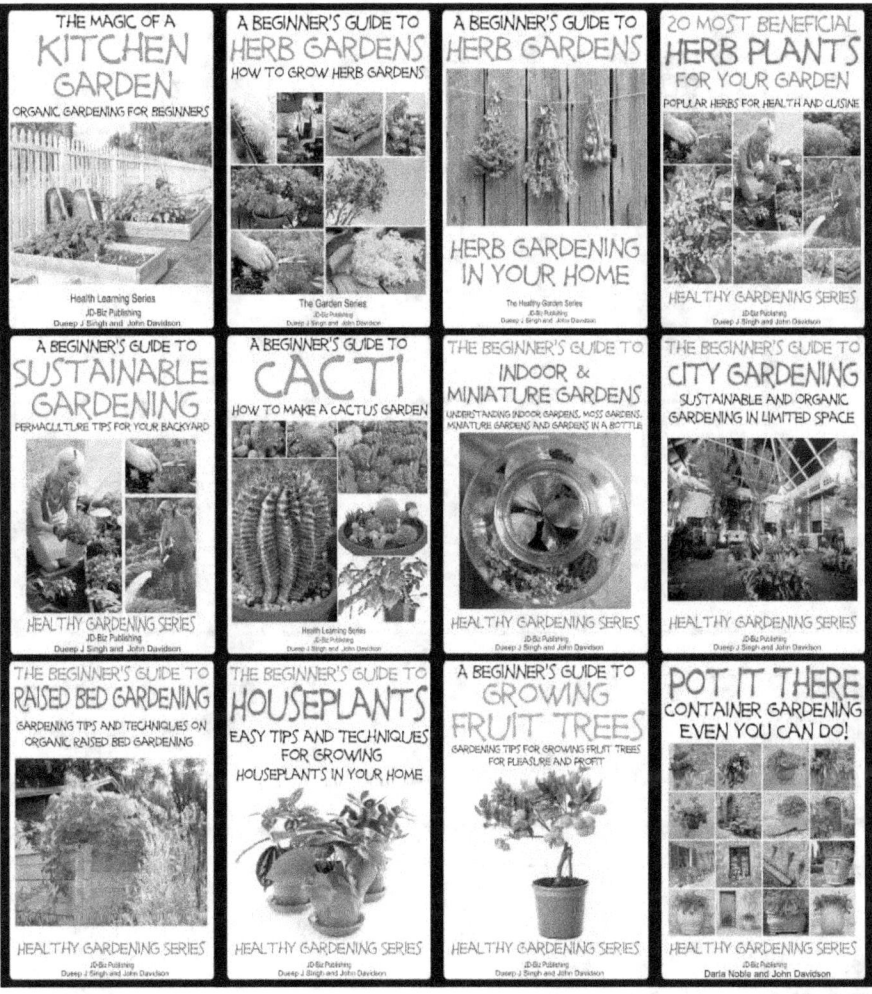

THE MAGIC OF GOOSEBERRIES FOR HEALTH AND BEAUTY	THE MAGIC OF YOGURT FOR COOKING AND BEAUTY	THE MAGIC OF LEMONS USING LEMONS FOR HEALTH AND BEAUTY	THE MAGIC OF CHILLIES FOR COOKING AND HEALING	THE MAGIC OF ONIONS ONIONS IN CUISINE TO CURE AND TO HEAL	THE MAGIC OF RADISHES TO CURE AND TO HEAL
THE MAGIC OF CARROTS TO CURE AND TO HEAL	THE HEALTH BENEFITS OF OREGANO FOR COOKING AND HEALTH	The Magic of MARIGOLDS Marigolds for health And Beauty	THE HEALTH BENEFITS OF CINNAMON	THE MAGIC OF COCONUTS FOR COOKING & HEALTH	THE MAGIC OF CLOVES FOR HEALING AND COOKING
THE MAGIC OF ASAFETIDA FOR COOKING AND HEALING	THE MAGIC OF NEEM MARGOSA TO HEAL	THE MAGIC OF SALT TO HEAL AND FOR BEAUTY	THE MAGIC OF POMEGRANATES FOR HEALTH AND BEAUTY	THE MAGIC OF DRY FRUIT AND SPICES REMEDIES AND RECIPES	THE HEALTH BENEFITS OF TURMERIC CURCUMIN FOR COOKING AND HEALTH
THE MAGIC OF ALOE VERA	THE MAGIC OF VEGETABLES ANCIENT HEALING REMEDIES AND TIPS	THE HEALTH BENEFITS OF ROSEMARY FOR COOKING AND HEALTH	THE MAGIC OF PEPPER & PEPPERCORNS FOR COOKING & HEALING	THE MAGIC OF MILK, BUTTER AND CHEESE FOR COOKING & HEALING	THE MAGIC OF CARDAMOMS FOR COOKING AND HEALTH
THE HEALTH BENEFITS OF BLACK CUMIN FOR COOKING AND HEALTH	THE MAGIC OF BASIL-TULSI TO HEAL NATURALLY	THE MAGIC OF SPICES FOR HEALTH AND CUISINE	THE MAGIC OF ROSES FOR COOKING AND BEAUTY	The Miraculous Healing Powers of GINGER	The Miracle of HONEY

Country Life Books

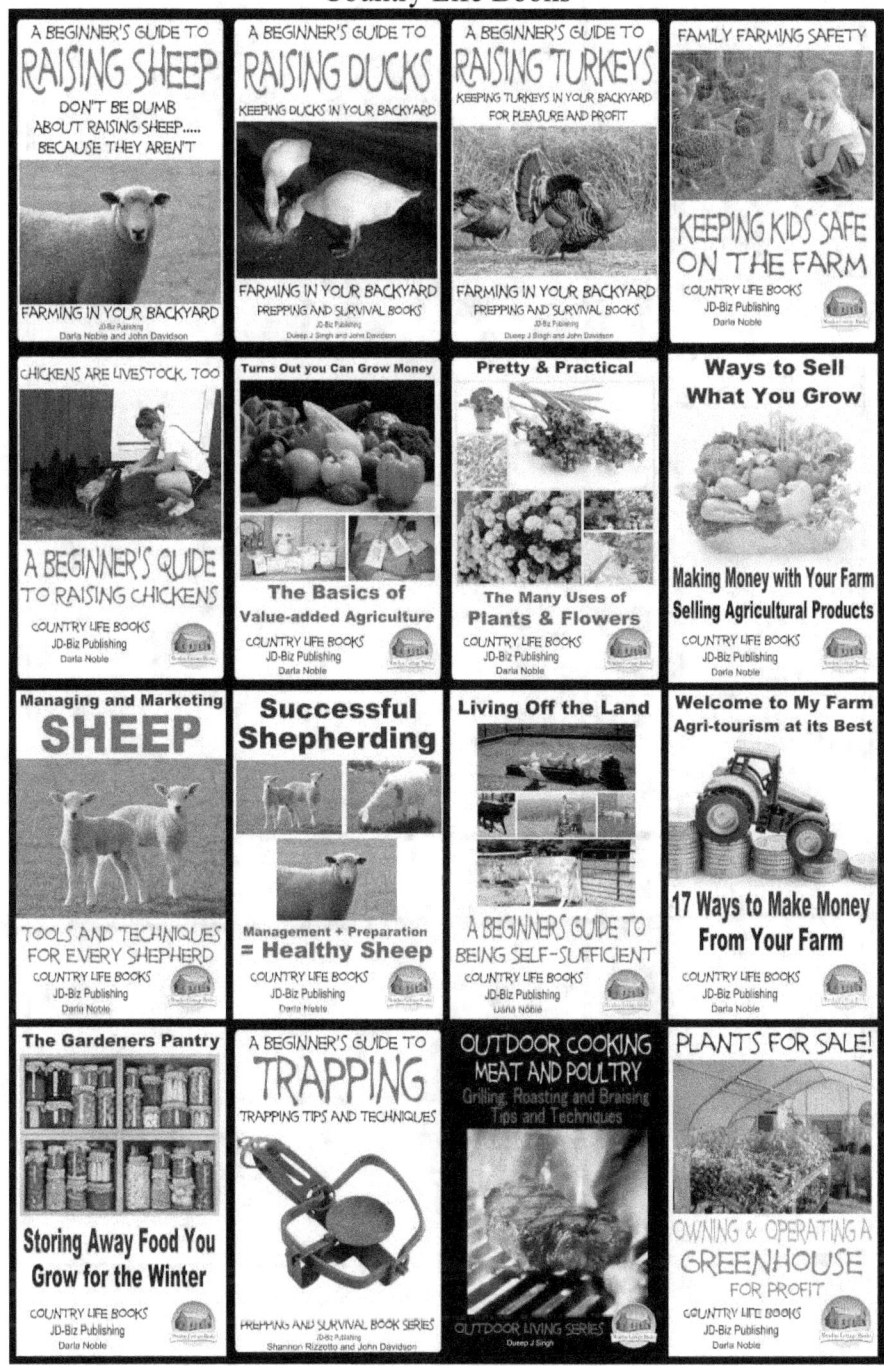

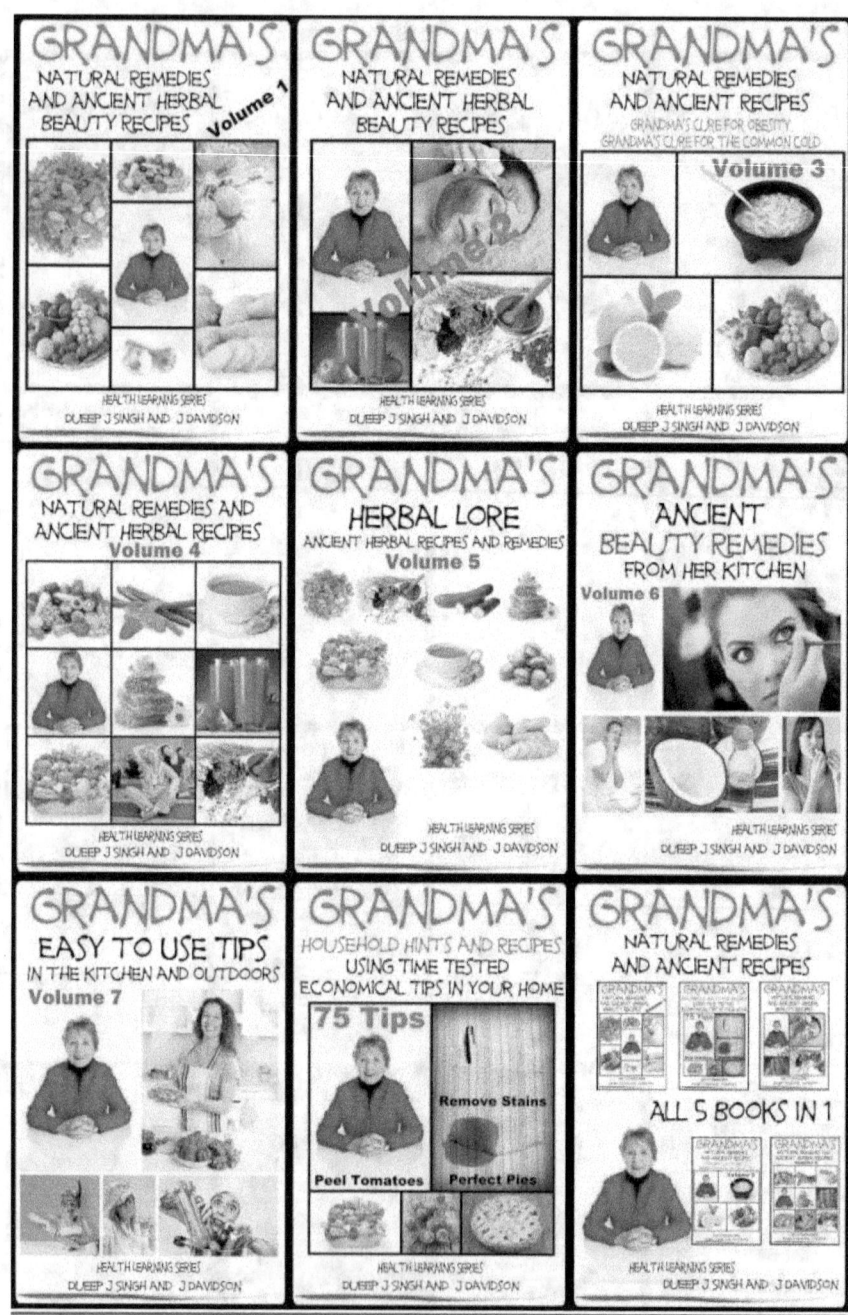

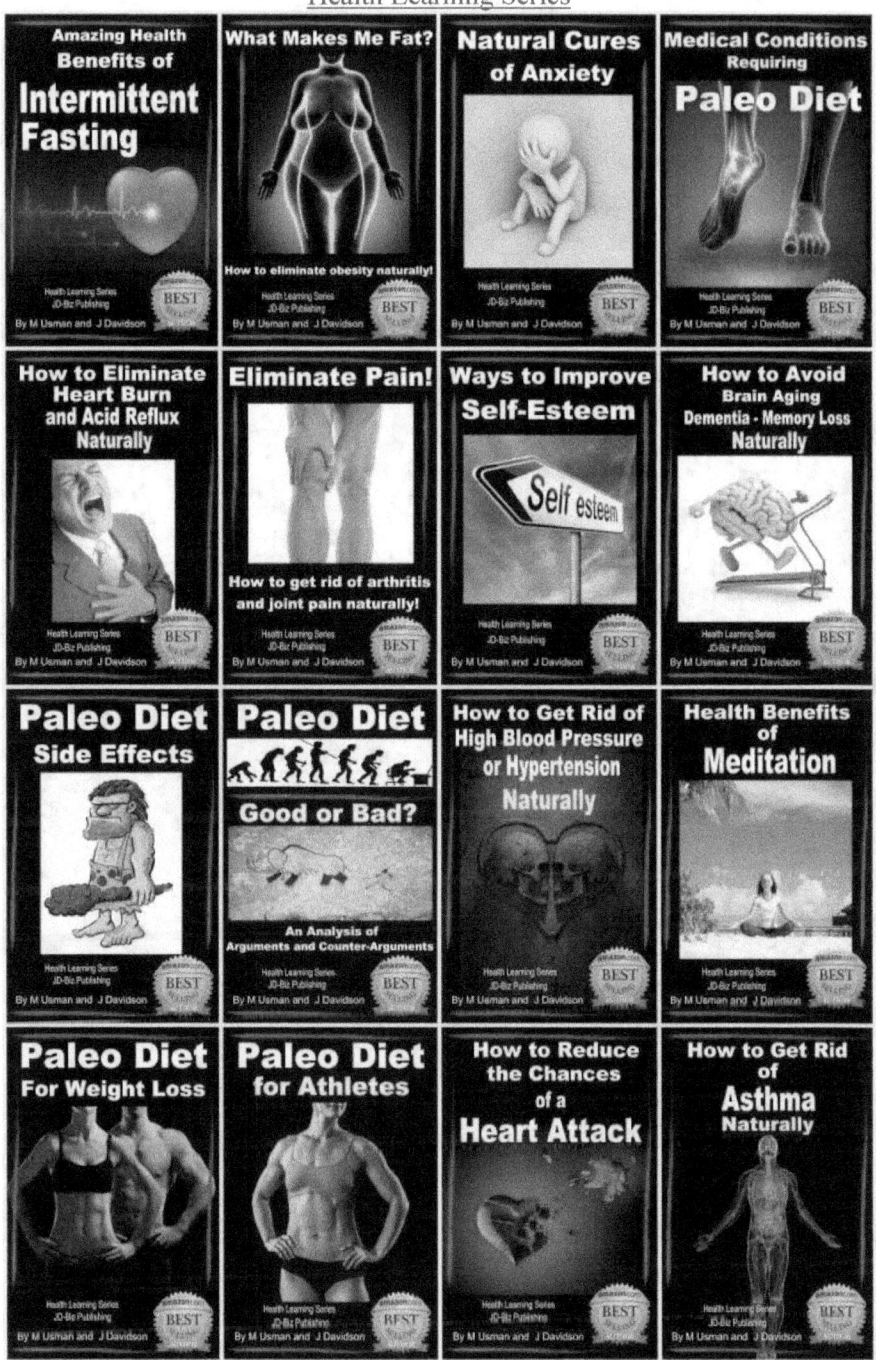

<u>Amazing Animal Book Series</u>

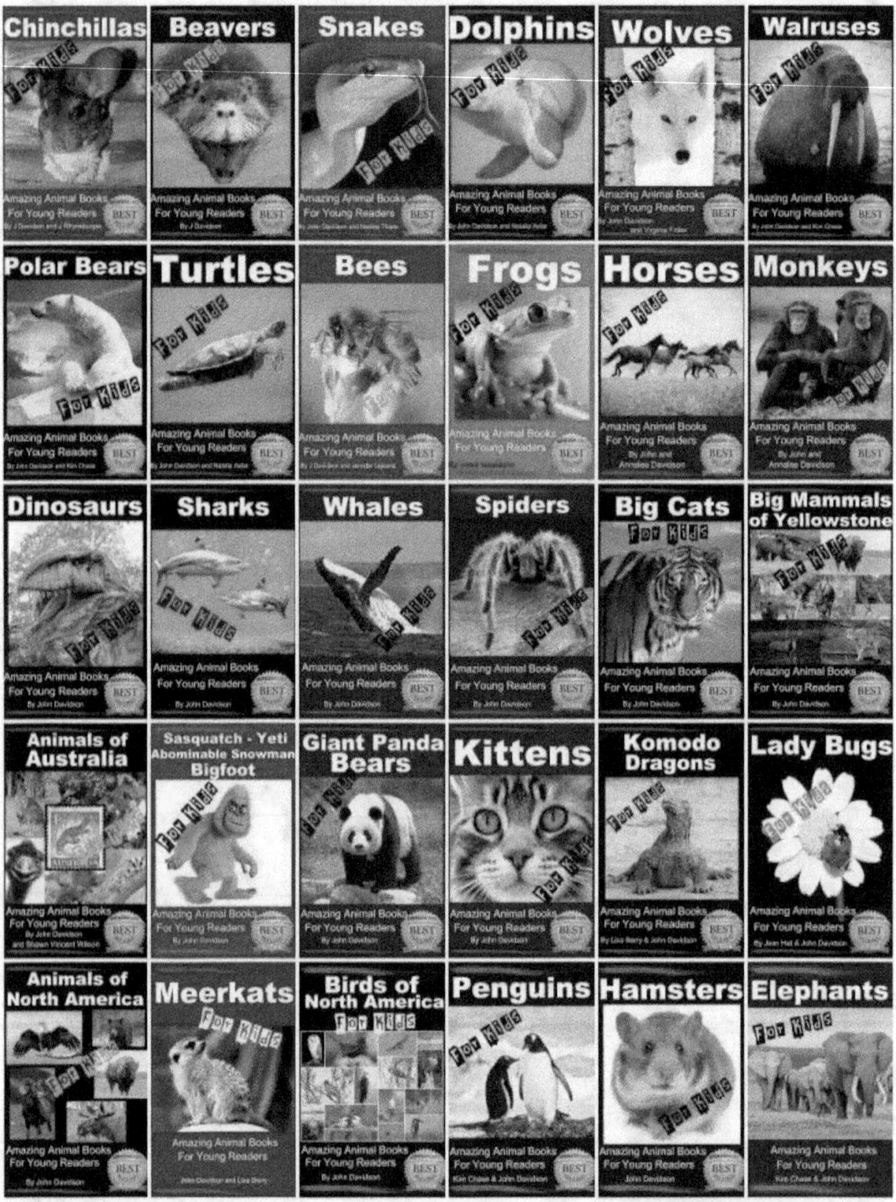

Learn To Draw Series

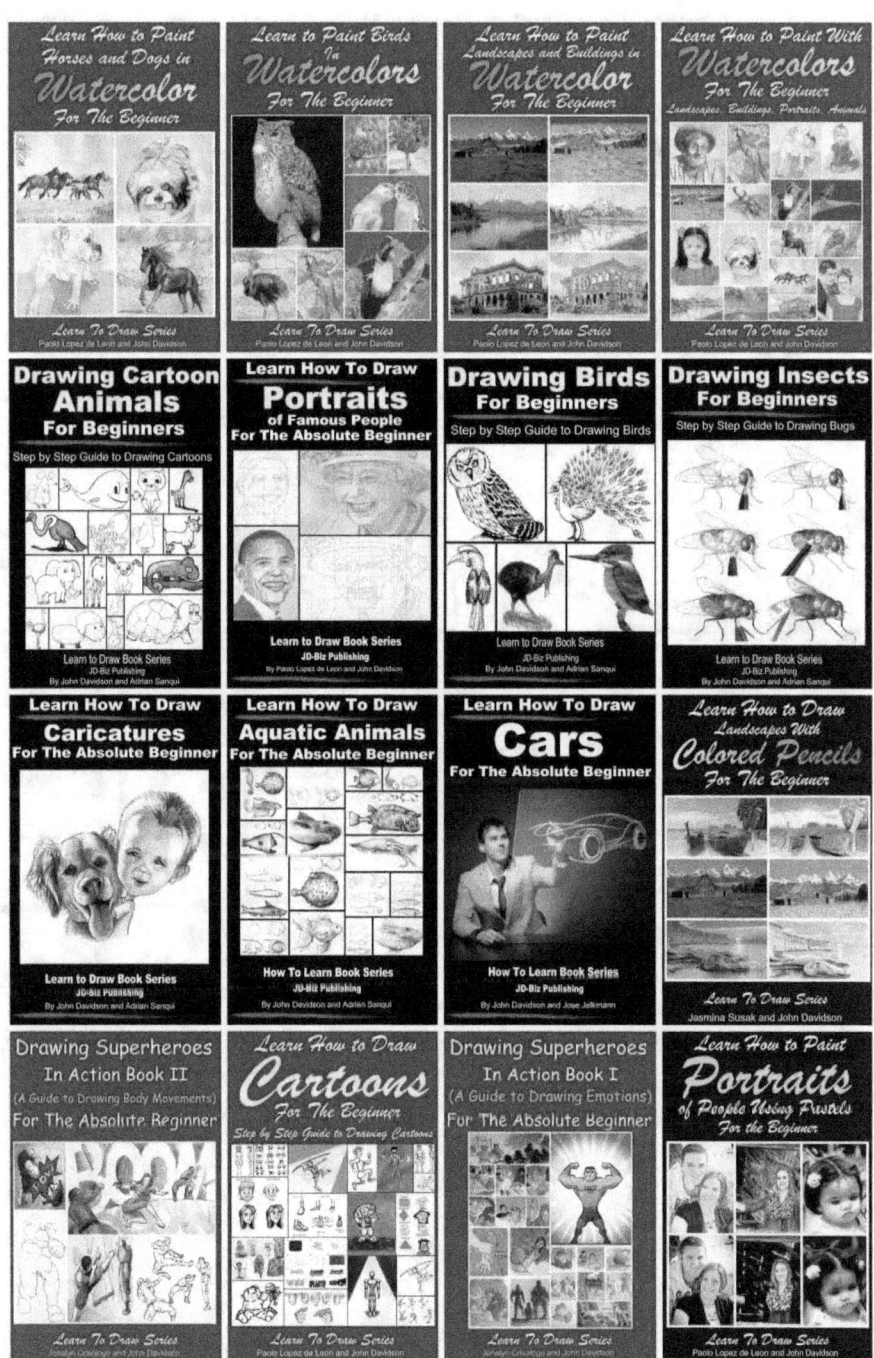

How to Build and Plan Books

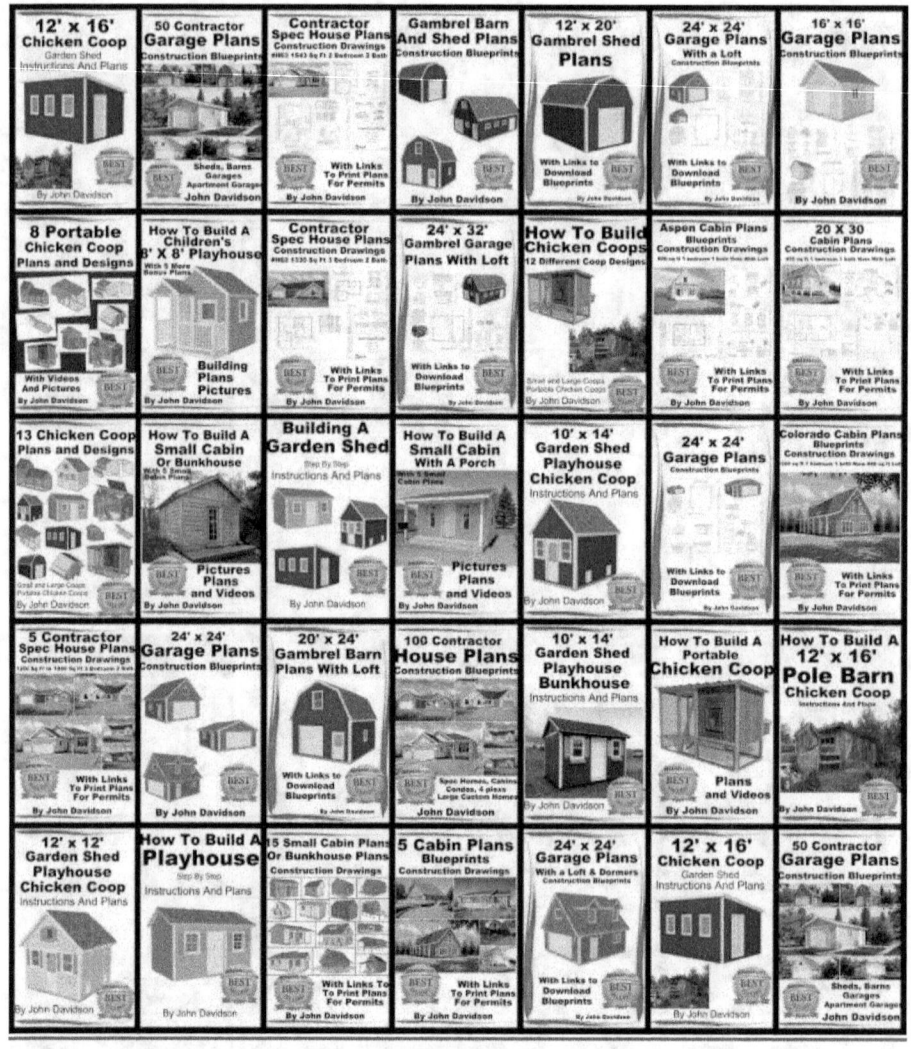

Entrepreneur Book Series

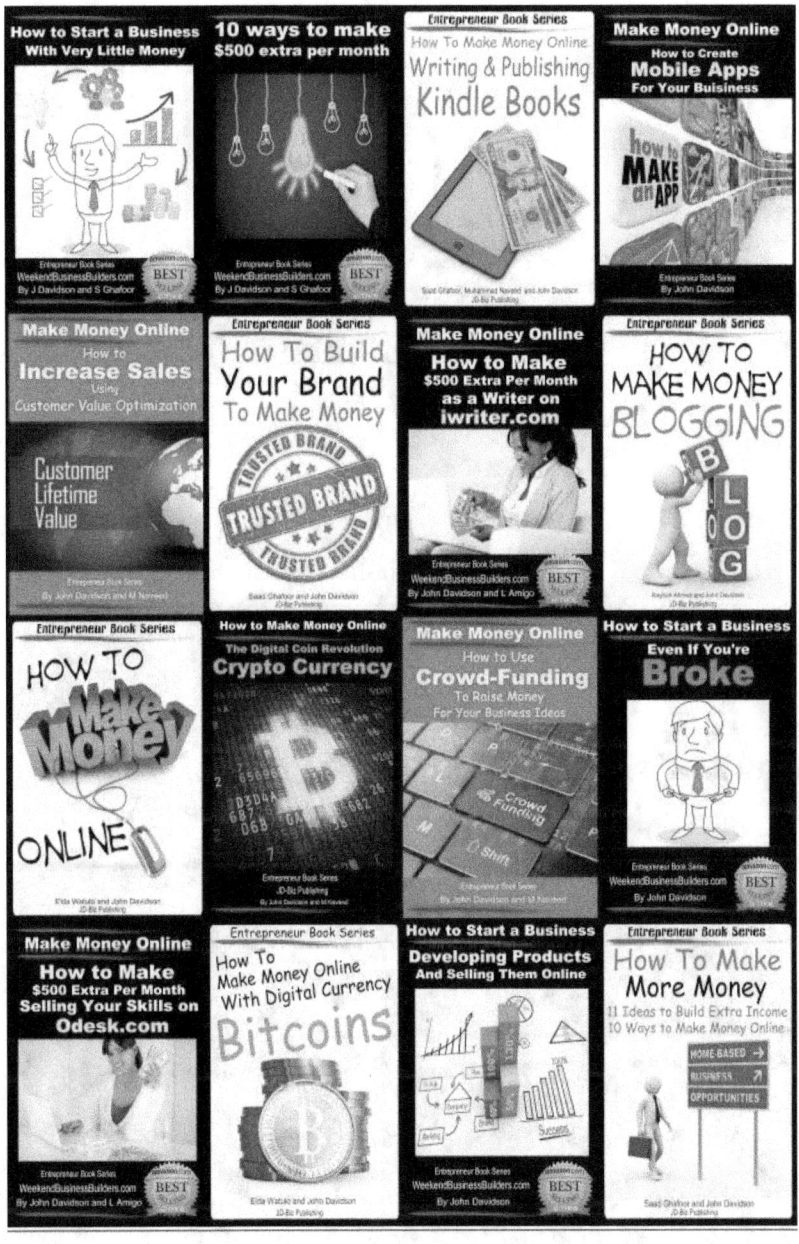

Publisher

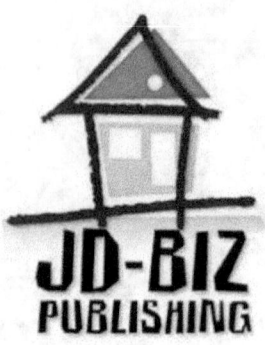

JD-Biz Corp

P O Box 374

Mendon, Utah 84325

http://www.jd-biz.com/

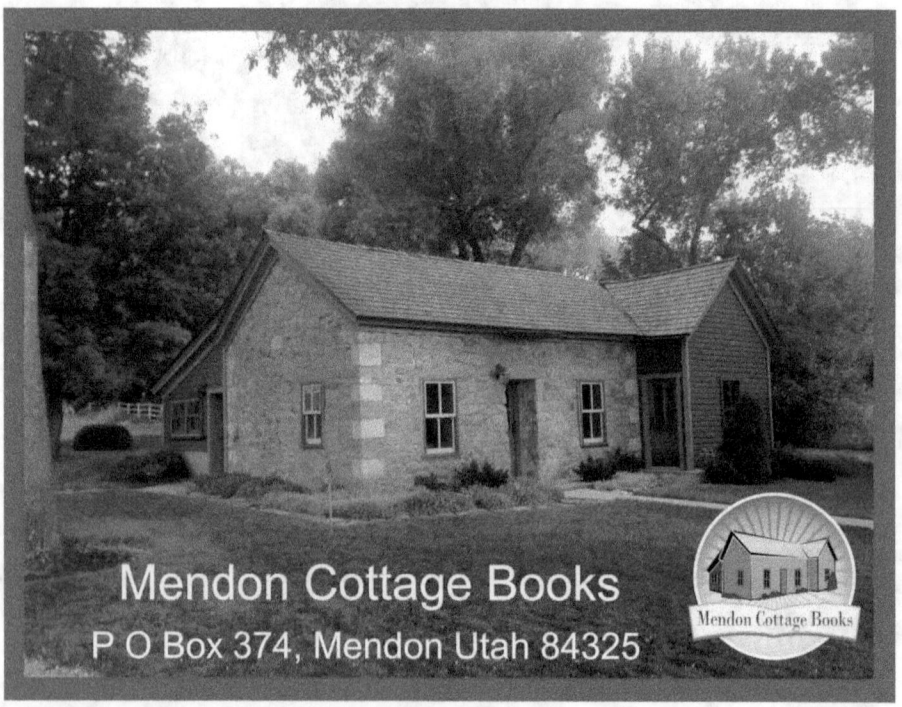